FOOD JOURNAL

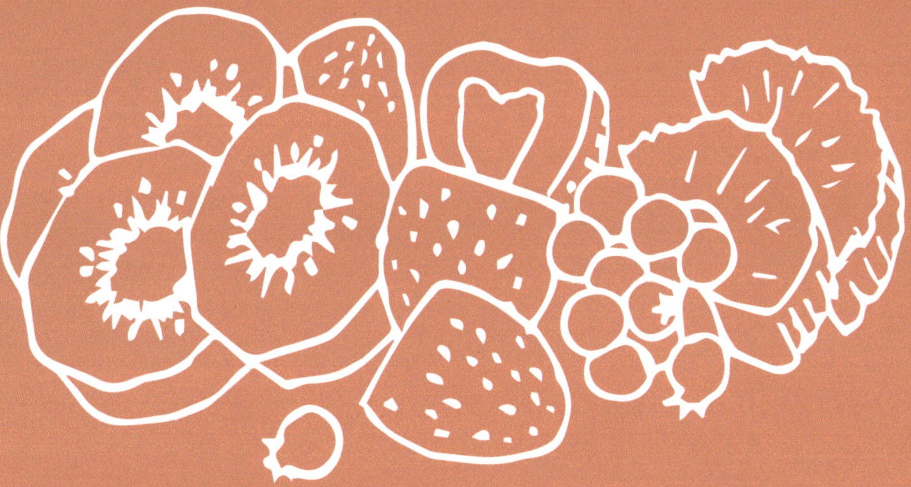

little
BLUEPRINT

little
BLUEPRINT
Empowering children. Training the brain.
WWW.LITTLEBLUEPRINT.COM

Made in the USA
Monee, IL
05 November 2026

67383068R00057